The Miracle of Breath

The Art of Breathing Well Learned from Ancient Eastern Medicine for Chronic Pain Rehabilitation, <u>Healing Illness</u>, Longevity, and More!

-- By Dr. Quang Do --

Copyright © 2021

TABLE OF CONTENT

INTRODUCTION

"For breath is life, and if you breathe well, you will live long on earth." - Sanskrit proverb

Let me start with a true story of how the miracles of breath saved a patient with pulmonary tuberculosis.

Dr. Vien Nguyen Khac, a doctor of modern medicine in Vietnam, was born in 1913. In 1942, he suffered from severe pulmonary tuberculosis. He was treated at Saint Hilaire du Touvet Hospital in Grenoble, Paris, France. In the mid-20th century, pulmonary tuberculosis had no cure as it does now. It was like a death sentence for those sick with the illness.

Within 6 years of treatment in Paris, France (from 1943-1948), Dr. Vien had to undergo many operations to treat pulmonary tuberculosis including 7 operations, cut 8 ribs, and the censor of the entire right lung and 1/3 left lung. His remaining breathing capacity was very low - only 1 liter. This is the lung capacity of a very weak person. According to the diagnosis of French doctors, he only had about 2 years to live. Many people thought he was not healthy enough to work at that time.

However, as a doctor, he did not accept lying down and waiting for death. He read in the resort library about oriental nutrition methods and he put all this knowledge together into developing a simple breathing exercise to cure himself. As a result, he lived for 50 years more than expected. He died in 1997 when he was 85 years old. Moreover, during those 50 years, he was still very healthy, still worked normally, wrote many books, and also traveled abroad many times. Dr. Vien overcame his illness and enjoyed a healthy life thanks to his breathing excercise practice.

That story may be hard to believe but it's true!

Dr. Vien said that, when sitting in lectures or in meetings, when others finished speaking, they often felt drowsy, and out of breath. However, he who was with only two-thirds of the lung structure was still comfortable and leisured. He revealed that in meetings or while waiting for someone, waiting for the bus, anywhere that he sat, it was then that he practiced the breathing exercise. Also, thanks to that breathing exercise, he slept very well, did not feel stressed, and did not get tired easily.

If you have never tried a breathing exercise, these tips in this book will help you overcome all obstacles to start practicing them. Dr. Vien's breathing exercises not only useful for young and healthy people but also help the sick, adults of all ages in particular the elderly and kids to strengthen their lungs and their immune systems to help them to cope better with the pandemic. Those exercises also help us reduce stress and sleep issues such as insomnia, which are common modern concerns.

Doctor Vien's breathing method is actually not something completely new. It is just a synthesis of qigong, meditation, yoga, tai chi, and nourishment derived from Eastern ancient practices. These practices were infused with modern respiratory physiology by a modern physician.

THE INCREDIBLE BENEFITS OF BREATHING

Modern research is showing us that a slight adjustment to the way we inhale and exhale can produce the same results as exercising. Such results include burning excess fat, slimming the body and abdomen, and rejuvenating internal organs. More so, this adjustment keeps the body supple, promotes longevity, cures the common cold, prevents snoring, and treats autoimmune diseases like asthma.

According to Oriental medicine, proper breathing and daily breathing exercises nourishes the kidneys, keeps the kidneys warm, and helps circulate blood effectively. This leads to the following benefits:

- Improving lung capacity
- Detox the body
- Better sleep quality
- Refreshed mind
- Prevention of depression and stress
- Controlled anxiety
- Prevention of health complications like kidney stones

- Regulation of blood pressure
- Regulation of heart rate
- Management of chronic pain
- Improvement of diabetes symptoms
- Strengthens resistance and enhances endurance of the body
- Increased longevity.

For those who have to lie in one place for a long time, the risk of lung infection is very high. The right breathing and breathing exercises will be a simple and effective way that patients can apply to prevent this. Breathing exercises not only help the patient reduce the risk of lung infections but will assist in reducing fatigue, reducing pain, sleeping better, and stimulating the body's self-healing mechanism.

For those who have just finished treating lung diseases, breathing exercises will help keep the lungs healthy. This is done by ensuring that the body has enough oxygen to feed the cells without burdening the lung. Therefore, the lungs can rest and quickly recover.

In addition, breathing exercises have many

advantages over other physical exercises. Such advantages include:

- It can be practiced anywhere, even in bed or while you're working.
- It can be used by people of all ages including from ages 5 to 100 years old. That means that the exercises can be utilized by the elderly, young children, busy people, people who are being treated for chronic diseases, if a person exercises regularly or not at all and so many other criteria.
- Application is inexpensive.
- There are no side effects.
- No equipment or machines are not necessary.
- Consumes a lot of calories despite being a simple exercise. Just 30 minutes of exercise per day also consumes an equal number of calories to structured exercising and working out for hours.
- Positive effects (refreshed body and mind, warmer hands and body, cure colds effectively, etc.) are felt immediately.

WHY WE SHOULD FOCUS ON EXERCISES TO INCREASE THE IMMUNE SYSTEM AND SELF-HEALING BODY?

Modern medicine believes that the change of environment including geography, toxic food, chemicals, viruses, bacteria, and more are the first causes of human diseases. But they account for only 10% of the causes of most diseases. The other factors that account for 90% of the causes of illness in the body are internal.

In everyday life, we have to work or study continuously. Because of prolonged stress and environmental pollution, our bodies have had to work too hard and have become more susceptible to disease.

Meanwhile, bacteria, viruses, and other pathogens are always changing into new and more complex versions. Modern vaccines, medicines, and therapies can only treat certain diseases and cannot promptly cure new diseases due to the rapid rate of transformation of pathogens. Therefore, instead of relying on modern medicines and therapies, it is essential that people take care of their immune system, practice healthy lifestyle habits such as exercise and diet, and have proper health care to lower the body's susceptibility to contracting diseases.

However, there are a few questions that need to be addressed:

- *Why, today, when we have modern health care are there are still many kinds of diseases?*
- *If we eat healthily, practice sports regularly, and get adequate health care, why are we still tired, stressed, anxious, sleepless, breathless, and very susceptible to disease?*
- *Besides eating healthily, resting adequately, regularly practicing sports, and practicing a proper health care routine, what have we missed?*

The answer to all of these questions is that almost all of us have skipped **practicing proper breathing**. People are always trying to increase the resistance and endurance of the body by spending a considerable amount of time in sports, going to the gym, or eating and using nutritional supplements. But we often forgot about the importance of good breathing.

All of us breathe – quite obviously - but most of us breathe unconsciously, and thus, most of us breathe improperly. So proper breathing is also a skill to learn and one which takes conscious effort.

THE POWER OF PROPER BREATHING

For thousands of years, ancient cultures have emphasized special breathing methods because they have been found to add value to a person's health and well-being. Oriental meditation, relaxation, and nourishing practices including yoga, qigong consider breathing as an integral part of the exercise.

Our life depends not only on meals, water, and sleep but also on our breath. We only eat 3-5 meals a day, but we breathe in, and out, and repeat this cycle twenty-five thousand (25,000) times per day. In addition to providing us with oxygen, breathing activates many physiological mechanisms in the body.

Nothing is as needed for our good health, happiness, and wellness as breath. As a species, however, humans have lost the ability to breathe correctly, with dire consequences. That's because most of us underestimate the importance of the breath. This is because we have been unconsciously breathing since we were born. So, we hardly pay much attention to the action even though while the average person can fast for 3 weeks, and not drink water for 3 days, this person can only hold his breath for about 3 minutes!

Breathe correctly by spending just 15 minutes a day practicing the simple breathing exercises. Remember that anyone can practice these exercises - from young children, adolescents, adults, the elderly, and patients. Even when you are young and healthy, do not forget to correct your breathing to stay healthy, prevent disease, promote alertness, and sleep well.

Having grasped the knowledge in this book based on thousands of years of medical texts and recent advanced research on correct breathing, body purification, psychology, biochemistry, and human physiology, you will never breathe the wrong way again.

No matter what you eat, how much exercise you do, or whether you are young or old, start breathing properly and practice breathing exercises now. Even if you are healthy, you will see its amazing effects.

HOW DOES YOUR BREATH HELP REJUVENATE YOUR CELLS?

The smallest components of our human body are cells. From cells that make up tissue, tissue creates organs and the organs that make up the complete body. As with solar panels, cells are always demanding to be fully charged and to be energized.

In addition to eating to regenerate cells' energy, breathing plays an important role because it will provide cells with oxygen. Breathing incorrectly deprives cells of oxygen, leading to a lack of energy. When there is a shortage of energy sources, the cell is imbalanced. This causes disturbances in essential activities like metabolism. Think of this analogy... When we get tired from physical labor, our bodies require rest and food to recharge this used energy. Not supplying the body with rejuvenating practice will harm overall health.

Cells work similarly. If there is not enough energy for a long time, the imbalance in cells can cause damage to tissues, contamination of blood, improper blood flow, and hiccups in the way the nervous system operates to name just a few ill effects. Eventually, this wears down cells and causes illness in different parts of the body.

When we breathe properly and practice breathing exercises, we get as much oxygen into our lungs as possible, so that the body and cells are not deprived of oxygen. At the same time, we expel as much carbon dioxide (CO2), a waste product, as possible out of the body. As a result, we reduce the toxic air mass in the lungs. That significantly increases the circulation of oxygen, the source of life for humans, in the bloodstream, and then can heal many health problems.

HOW TO BREATHE IN THE RIGHT WAY

Breathing is classified as more important and more effective than macrobiotic methods. Modern science also recognizes that all process of the body requires oxygen. The lack of oxygen will make the body tired, impaired memory, create mental sluggishness, and promote the development of depression and stress. From the past up to now, those who breathe properly have always had improved mental, emotional, and physical health.

All of us know how to breathe properly from birth, but as we grow, we forget it. Observing children under 2 years old, we can see that the abdomen rises and falls with each breath. But for adults, the movement of the respiratory is mainly on the chest area.

This difference is because when people begin to walk and working steadily with two legs, lung activity begins to shift from the lower half of the lung upwards. This causes the lungs to not function as efficiently. Therefore, we don't breathe at the full capacity as we will not inhale enough air into the lungs. The body is supplied with less oxygen with each breath in.

In most cases, ***the wrong breathing is not due to insufficient inhalation, but insufficient exhalation***. If we do not exhale all the air from our lungs, we will reuse the carbon dioxide (CO_2) that remains in the lungs. This decreases the distribution of oxygen (O_2) to our body.

Removing all of the air from the lungs creates space for new fresh air to enter your lungs. If we exhale lightly (shallow breathing), only a portion of the air in the lungs is removed. The remaining air prevents as much new fresh air from entering the lungs as if possible. This means that there is no air metabolism, which gradually limits or shrinks the lower lung sac in a process called atelectasis. The lungs lose their capacity to expand. If we pay attention to exhaling all the old air at the bottom of the lung (deep breathing), the new air entering the bottom of the lung causes the air exchange in the basal air sacs to be performed. This causes the lungs to expand and thus, perform healthily. The amount of air (O_2) and (CO_2) passing through the lungs promotes healthy air metabolism and comprehensively improves lung function.

The best way to breathe to push all the air out of the lungs is called deep breathing. It is performed by moving the diaphragm and abdominal muscles. As a result, it is also called abdominal breathing. If we pay attention to exhaling all the old air at the bottom of the lungs (deep breathing), the new air entering the bottom of the lung causes the air exchange in the basal air sacs to be performed. This causes the lungs to expand more, leading to an increased lung capacity.

Breathing movements are performed with a muscular system that includes:

- The diaphragm, which is the horizontal muscle between the chest and abdomen. This is the main part that facilitates breathing. It divides the upper surface arch of the chest adjacent to the heart and the lungs, and the lower surface adjacent to the liver and abdominal cavity, including the digestive organs, stomach, intestines, and internal organs.

- When the diaphragm is lowered, the lower rib cage expands. At the same time, the muscles attached to the ribs pull up the ribs. The chest expands in two directions: vertical and horizontal.

- The lower part of the chest expands the most because it consists of soft parts. The diaphragm is the base of the thorax, and the anterior flanks are the cartilage. The upper part of the thorax is also enlarged, but less because this is the hard part, consisting of ribs that pull from the spine to the sternum.

- When the diaphragm is lowered, the internal organs in the abdomen are pushed down. The abdomen swells up. At that time, the air is sucked in so there is a bulge. When the diaphragm is raised, the air is expelled, the internal organs in the abdomen are pulled, and the abdomen shrinks so there is a movement of the abdomen to exhale.

In short, breathing properly requires the following to occur:

- Inhalation: Abdominal bulge.

- Exhalation: Abdominal contraction.

- Rhythm: Regular, calm, slow. All breathing movements are normal following the body's natural rhythm.

In the case that the mind can focus on the breath, one more factor is needed:

Exhale more slowly than inhaling (as opposed to normal, unconscious natural breathing).

Abdominal breathing not only helps the body breathe enough oxygen nourishing the cells, but it also helps to burn excess fat by using the muscles in the abdomen as above. In addition, according to Oriental Medicine, the abdomen has 8 meridians and 1 vessel going through it. These are all important channels of the body. Breathing through the abdomen helps to activate the operating channels. Of course, it also helps to regulate oxygen and carbon dioxide levels, whereby the body becomes circulating and significantly improves health.

DETAILED INSTRUCTIONS FOR PROPER BREATHING EXERCISES

Dr. Vien's breathing exercise can be briefly described as follows:

- Deeply exhale and tighten your stomach as much as possible

- Abdominal bulge inhalation

- Two shoulders remain motionless

- The limbs remain relaxed

- Breath slowly, steadily, and deeply

- Focus on the exhale and inhale

This exercise can be done:

- Standing or lying down

- Wherever

- Anytime!

Without further ado, here are some breathing exercises that increase resistance, heal, increase endurance, live a long, healthy life, and more.

<u>Exercise 1: Abdominal breathing with a 1:1 inhalation - exhalation ratio</u>

This is the easiest exercise for beginners. This is also an exercise for young, healthy, and busy people who do not have much time to practice. This is also the exercise that Dr. Vien often applied and many people have followed. Here are the steps:

- **Step 1**: Sit in a chair or lie on a bed with your back straight, and your arms and shoulders relaxed. Do not move your shoulders. Imagine you are holding a cup of hot water to help you do so. You need to inhale, then exhale and blow out gently to blow it down. Slowly and gently. When your stomach is tightened as much as possible, stop blowing. Then gently expand your stomach to breathe in through your nose. When your stomach bulges up, pause for a moment and exhale. Continue to exhale while tightening the stomach muscles in as much as possible. Practice this for 5-10 minutes then rest.

- **Step 2**: After getting used to the abdominal contraction (exhale) and bulge (inhale), there's no need to let air through the mouth anymore. Then just breathe in and out through your nose. Practice breathing as much as possible in the following postures: lying on your back (with two legs folded), lying on your stomach, lying on your side, crawling on all fours, kneeling, and standing with arms crossed. While walking on the street, sitting on a bike, or motorbike, sitting on the bus, waiting for someone else, or whenever you feel stressed, do this exercise a few times.

Benefits of Exercise 1

- Makes the most of the lung capacity. The lifting of the diaphragm helps to exchange thoracic capacity, increases the maximum lung capacity, and helps the internal organs to be massaged according to the breath and the nervous system relax.

- Can be practiced at any time and place.

- Suitable for all ages, especially children, or those who are busy with work and who have to spend a lot of time taking care of the home, children.

The essence of this exercise is breathing properly - abdominal breathing. You can practice this breathing exercise while studying, working, sitting on the bus, waiting for someone, sitting in a meeting, anywhere... You will not lose any time but can have achieved nearly 100% of the effectiveness of lung capacity with this breathing exercise.

Exercise 2: Abdominal breathing with a 1:2 inhalation-exhalation ratio

This breathing exercise is similar to **Exercise 1**. However, you extend the exhale twice as long as the inhalation.

Benefits of Exercise 2:

- The same benefits as in **Exercise 1**.

- Besides, extending the exhalation time will help us fully exhale residue air in the lungs, maximize the lung clearance, increase maximum lung capacity for the most effective inhalation, increase the amount of oxygen we inhale more for our lungs, and body.

Exercise 3: 4-Phased Breathing (inhalation, breath-holding, exhalation, breath-holding)

- **Step 1**: Inhale slowly and gently through the nose for as long as you can tolerate, while bulging your abdomen.

- **Step 2**: Hold your breath.

- **Step 3**: Exhale slowly, gently, and long, and at the same time your stomach will fill all the way.

- **Step 4**: Hold your breath for the same amount of time as in **Step 2**.

At the beginning of practice, the practitioner can use a count of 1, 2, 3, 4, 5 in each phase. Then this person can increase the time by counting to 7, 8, 9, 10.

The difficulty of this exercise is to inhale to the maximum, hold the breath for a long time, and then exhale slowly. You need to hold your breath for so long as possible but also keep your muscles relaxed, and your expression calm. Practitioners need to practice slowly, gradually increasing each breath time up to the maximum.

Benefits of Exercise 3:

- The same benefits as in **Exercise 1**.

- Significantly increases the benefits of **Exercise 1** by having more time to hold your breath, retaining more oxygen in the body, and extending the time to fully exhale residue in the lungs. Emptying the lungs maximally increases maximum lung capacity for the most effective inhalation. This exercise can also be used in preparation for practicing the intensive exercise (**Exercise 5**).

Exercise 4: Breathe while walking

This exercise combines breathing practice with walking and is most suitable for the elderly suffering from a health condition. While walking, combine the action with gentle and deep abdominal breathing using following the formula:

- 4 breaths in while expanding the abdomen

- 2 breathes, held in

- 8 breaths out while tightening the stomach muscles

The time of each breath is usually 3-5 seconds, depending on how slow the breathing rhythm. You can walk fast or slow, or short or long distance depending on the ability of each person while doing this. The exercise will be more effective when walking in a well-ventilated, place supplied with fresh air, and when the practitioner has a relaxed and comfortable spirit.

<u>**Exercise 5: Intensive breathing exercise**</u>

This is an intensive exercise and also the one that will gain you the most benefits. After you get used to the above exercises, try doing this in-depth breathing exercise.

If the 4 above breathing exercises only help you maximize your lung capacity, then *this exercise will help you get all the miracles of breath mentioned at the beginning of this book*. So if you're not too busy, don't forget to spend 15-30 minutes daily practicing this breathing exercise. Let me remind you of the benefits you will get from this specific breathing exercise:

- Maximize lung capacity
- Detox the body
- Better sleep quality
- Refreshed mind
- Prevention of depression and stress
- Controlled anxiety
- Prevention of health complications like kidney stones

- Regulation of blood pressure

- Regulation of heart rate

- Management of chronic pain

- Improvement of diabetes symptoms

- Strengthens resistance and enhances endurance of the body

- Increased longevity.

This exercise combines inhalation, breath-holding and exhalation using the following formula:

- Inhalation: 3 counts (to enlarge belly and chest to full size)

- Hold your breath: 3 counts

- Exhale: 6 counts

- Hold your breath: 2 counts

- Continue to exhale: 3 counts

- Hold your breath: 1 count

- Continue to exhale: 5-10 counts to let all the air in your abdomen and chest out, depending on your body.

• 1 deep inhalation. Then inhale and exhale according to **Exercise 1** to relax.

The time of each count is usually 3-5 seconds, depending on how slow the breathing rhythm.

<u>Note:</u>

• Be aware of your breath, feel your abdomen expand and contract, and breathe actively - CONTROL your breath.

• In this exercise, for the first 3 counts, try to inhale as much as possible.

• As explained in the previous part of this book, the wrong breathing is often not due to insufficient inhalation but insufficient exhalation. So once you get used to this exercise, exhaling as much as possible. Increase the number of breaths out during exercise gradually.

• At the end of the exercise is when all the air in the abdomen and chest will be exhaled entirely.

The more you exhale to the end, the more residue air will be squeezed out.

- Always keep the back straight while keeping the whole body relaxed.

When all the air in the abdomen and chest will be exhaled entirely, it creates a strong pressure that causes full inhalation. Then a new amount of oxygen-rich air entering into each of your cells to take out the dirt, and put in new air to create a clean, circulating, oxygen-filled environment inside. This helps speed up the process of blood circulation. This is the principle and meaning of practical breathing.

For best results, do this exercise at least 20-30 times a day. Elderly people lying in bed can be done 40-60 times/day.

COMMON MISTAKES MADE WHEN PRACTICING BREATHING EXERCISES

I knew about the true story of Dr. Vien and breathing exercises a long time ago and tried breathing exercises before but was lazy with the practice. It was not until I was ill and suffered a mild stroke that I began to try breathing exercise (**Exercise 5**) seriously. The first few days, when I completed practicing, I felt very tired, not refreshing. After observing myself, I noticed that I made the following mistakes:

Error 1: Tightening my body a lot while practicing breathing. I found myself tense when I practiced. I tightened my neck muscles, shoulder muscles, back muscles, abdominal muscles, glutes, thigh muscles, and more as I inhaled, held my breath, and expelled air. This took more energy than breathing. My breathing was therefore short, and ineffective, both draining my body and getting me tired quickly.

Error 2: My inhales and exhales were too hard. I inhaled and exhaled so hard that every time I practiced active breathing, everyone around me heard it. When first practicing, a breath is often very crude, without coherence, flexibility, and lightness.

GENERAL NOTES FOR CORRECTLY PRACTICING BREATHING EXERCISES

Practicing the 5 breathing exercises outlined above requires that you follow specific procedures for maximum effectiveness. They include:

- As you breathe, take a deep breath and pay attention to your nose.

- Breathe in gently, feeling the airflow into your nose. Gently bulge your abdomen.

- When holding your breath, gently hold your breath through your nose. Notice that when you hold your breath there, you are holding my breath everywhere else. For example, check to see if your neck is stiff, your teeth are clenched, your shoulders are hunched, or your legs are sticking to the floor. If you feel strain in other parts of your body, immediately relax.

- When you exhale, simply exhale through your nose. There was no need to use the full-body strength to expel air. When I first started training, I often tightened my abdominal muscles to exhale. Gradually when I managed to control my breathing, I no longer had much abdominal contraction.

- Always keep your back straight. Don't stick out your chest. This is very important. When you exercise well, there will be a strong flow of energy running down your spine to your brain. Sitting bent or hunched over will prevent this energy flow, hamper your breathing and decrease your mental concentration. Therefore, the key to breathing comfortably and effectively is back comfort. Because the two sides of the spine are two energy flows, there are nerves and many acupuncture points that control all activities in the body. When the back is straight and comfortable, the energy in the body can be circulated for a clear and healthy mind.

- If you have trouble keeping your back straight and comfortable, lie down and breathe (instead of sitting and breathing).

WHAT ARE THE SIGNS THAT YOU HAVE PRACTICED CORRECTLY?

- When you fix common mistakes and practice correctly, you will find the practice of breathing softer.

- You will feel an overall improvement in wellness.

- You will feel more refreshed after each practice.

- After each breath, you will feel a stream of energy - warm air runs down the spine up the brain and to each finger and toes. When done, the body will feel warmer.

After I had a stroke, I just wanted to complete the exercise quickly and be well. But it took patience and consistency. Now, I feel a healthier body, a refreshed mind, and want to continue. It's like eating a portion of delicious food, you will want to eat more. For me, practicing breathing exercise (**Excercise 5**) 60 to 100 times per day becomes comfortable and refreshing. This is signs that the practice is on the right track.

The best practice time is in the morning when you first wake up. When you wake up, before getting out of bed, just lie down and practice **Exercise 5** for 5-10 times. This will help the body and mind have the necessary warm-up before preparing to work for the new day.

Besides, during other times of the day, you can practice it anytime.

For Dr. Vien, he always practiced breathing exercises before going to bed and in the morning when he started to wake up. If he ever felt tired (after an hour), he would stop working to meditate and practice breathing exercises.

Practicing proper breathing every day combined with a proper diet and rest will bring you great health to study, work, and enjoy life!

CONCLUSION

Thank you for making it to the end of this book. I am very happy to know that now you will know how to breathe properly and these miracle breathing exercises to heal all your health problems.

It doesn't take long to see results. Try breathing exercises today, you will see their amazing effects. I wish all my readers a healthy and happy life!

And please please leave an honest review of what you thought of this book! It will help me out a ton!!!

Thank you!